Pennies from Heaven

A Personal Experience of Providing Live-in Care with a Family Member or Friend with Dementia

Elisabeth Webb-Hooper

Published by

MELROSE BOOKS

An Imprint of Melrose Press Limited
St Thomas Place, Ely
Cambridgeshire
CB7 4GG, UK
www.melrosebooks.co.uk

FIRST EDITION

Cover by Melrose Books

ISBN	**978-1-912333-00-4 Paperback**
epub	**978-1-912333-01-1**
mobi	**978-1-912333-02-8**

Printed and bound in Great Britain by:
Lightning Source UK Ltd, Chapter House, Pitfield
Kiln Farm, Milton Keynes, MK11 3LW

To my darling Pops,
I love you always

Acknowledgements

There are several people who I really want thank for their help throughout my time in writing *Pennies From Heaven*.

Firstly, my darling husband and soulmate, Jason, who has gone over and above in his exceptional caring role and support with my father. My two children for their love and understanding to a dearest Pops.

To Neil, Mike, Tom and Ken for always being a good friend to Dad.

To Rodger and Leah, you have been exceptional support to us all. Thank you from the bottom of my heart.

To Adam, Angela, Nam and Sabina, you are truly friends for ever, and thank you from Pops.

To Verline, Nikki and Maria for your help when we needed it.

To all my friends who were there for me Pam, Peter(Bro), Karen, Shan, Sue, Linda, Michelle and Hameeda. Too many to write here, but I love you all for being there when you were needed.

A huge thank you to Claire for advice with Carewatch and to Aunty Pam, Julia and Maria for making Pops smile over a Danish pastry!

Thank you also to SSAFA, Alzheimer's Association, Carewatch and all carers and GPs who were there for us all.

Without your help, none of this would have been possible.

For Leah Ashby

During the publishing period of this book, our dear friend and mentor, Leah Ashby, sadly passed away.

Leah was special, dynamic, and without her strength and great support, over and above her field of duty, none of what we achieved would have been possible.

Leah was found by myself and husband in quite a unique set of events as I searched for help with getting support and advice to get Pops home from hospital after him being there for far too long. The circumstances were way out of our control as decision makers and social workers were away, and the day of Dad coming home seemed a real distant possibility; it was heartbreaking.

At the time, we found a really helpful advocate from the Alzheimer's Association who did come to our first hospital meeting to plan Dad's future, but she told us she was actually leaving for a new job role. We were heartbroken, that day, as we were told by all concerned that Dad could not come home. My POA was ignored. I was given Leah's phone number who would take on our case.

It was to be the best thing that could ever have happened to us all. After my prompt phone call, not being a person to let the grass grow under their feet, and having a long chat with Leah, our prayers had been answered. Leah was amazing. Her voice, her gorgeous accent made you feel calm and relaxed; she was a pocket rocket dynamo from the very first moment. I met Leah and she met Alex and all the family. We loved her, we felt safe. Leah was extremely knowledgeable and powerful. In fact, if she didn't know a small detail of case law, she would find out imminently. She challenged the top people when we knew they had given incorrect answers saying we couldn't cope and Dad could never come home. We proved everyone who said this wrong, and this is the reason for my book.

If you have a dementia-related illness, and it is manageable and practical to be nursed with the correct help and direction in your own home, with your loved ones around you, you should be allowed to do so.

It is a difficult time and a hard process for all concerned, but if it is the desire and last wish of anyone, then this should, and must be, respected.

Future Publications by Liz Hooper
Rainbows and Butterflies

Contents

Chapter 1
The early stages, with or without diagnosis

Personal experience

The early signs to observe with dementia are spotting unusual behaviour, such as perhaps putting items in strange places and forgetting where you have put them, or being unable to retain very basic information. Many of us can be oblivious to the early signs, especially when you live close to someone and their behaviour becomes 'normal'.

My father suffered a small TIA – transient ischaemic attack – in other words, a mini-stroke. From early visits to the memory clinic, it can be a very frightening and lonely experience as much for loved ones looking after a precious family member as it is for those suffering with the condition. The most important thing is to get help as soon as possible when you feel there is a cause for concern. A visit to the GP is crucial, as the earlier a person is seen and diagnosed the better. This can be a difficult time as very often, dementia sufferers will be in denial; however, there is a way forward and it is so important to get things right to help protect our loved ones.

Help is available and that is why I have decided to write this book. I have learned the good, bad and the ugly and want to share all of this with others to enable people to make the correct decisions and be very aware of the care system available. Most of my experience has been good, although tinged with bad and the bad has caused so much unnecessary stress. I want to make others aware of how best to deal with issues that arise and not to feel isolated, or embarrassed to ask for help.

Basic things to look out for

Sometimes people can hallucinate and perhaps think they see shadows or things moving – this can be a small crack in a wall or hole and is known as "sundown syndrome". A shiny surface or road can look like water or flooding and can cause alarm.

Many people suffering vascular dementia forget where they are and can look lost and confused. It is important to try and ensure they are not left alone for reasons of safety.

Time and days all roll into one for sufferers. In my case, vascular dementia caused the whole family to be involved – when it was the very early hours of morning and hearing the television or radio on was almost like reliving my teenage days, except it was a role reversal. Vascular dementia sufferers may think it is daytime when in fact it is two or three o'clock in the early hours of the morning. The problem comes with there being no persuasion that it is night time and this causes huge frustration as I and my husband found out, as your loved one does not understand. People read articles telling you to keep calm. It is not so easy to keep calm when you are tired and you want to go to sleep as you have work and a family to care for the following day whereas your loved one can sleep all day, and this is the problem.

When dementia has been diagnosed, make sure you tell others as there is nothing worse than someone feeling lost and confused and people not understanding why. Do this discreetly, as although dementia sufferers do seem to not always be aware of what people are talking about around them, they actually often are and it is very rude to make this common mistake. Reassurance is important. There are fantastic societies to help people with various groups running days with singing for the brain and photographic nostalgic times, The Alzheimer's Society and locally run groups. The most important point is to know and understand the person's previous lifestyle and use memory joggers such as photographs, as many times, dementia sufferers can go back way in the past so there is no point in just looking at a couple of years ago. Also, music, music, music is a great help. Look back to their family, their parents and siblings, friends and work colleagues. Find items of interest, but also be very aware that sufferers can end up destroying photographs, so make sure there are copies as there is sometimes a complete lack of understanding that these items are precious.

One of the worst things is the fear people have, and friends which were once so close can seem to drift away and not seem to care, but often they just can't deal with a close friend changing. I have had this experience, and it does make you feel that you can be quite alone and isolated. It is also partly why I needed to write this book. My husband and some close friends have been amazing with my father, yet some of my father's friends have drifted. It has to be understood that these people may find it difficult to come to terms with their once-active friend who they laughed and joked with and who has changed so dramatically. This, however, doesn't need to be the case, as re-visiting good times can be a very positive thing and turn on a glimmer of light!

Positive thinking!
Fill the world of the dementia sufferer with things they love.

For myself this has been music, music and more music, followed by chocolate, cake and trifle. Photographs, books, letters and memorabilia which can turn a small spark into a fireball of delight! It is so uplifting to the spirit of your loved one and yourself. If there is a fabulous friend, get them to visit and talk about lovely times from the past. My father was a guardsman, also a Ballroom and Latin American dance teacher, a Gold member with the Imperial Society of Teachers of Dancing, teaching until four years prior to becoming ill. He also has some good friends who provide inspiration. Remember, just a small thing can have such a positive outcome!

Chapter 2
Dark times

The beginning of a whole new world of care!

In June 2014 after a fall, Dad went into hospital. He was there for almost four weeks. At the first of what would be many hospital meetings, it was decided that a care package would be the best way forward to help my father live at home. We, my husband, cousin and myself, were to have a meeting with a GP, social worker and a member of Community Health Team. The GP was very good, explaining the way that vascular dementia can be likened to the M4 with some smaller routes blocked-off. It was agreed that Dad was to have four carers per day. This was going to be a whole new experience for us all, but what we did insist on was that care should be kept to a small number of carers to ensure familiarity to my Dad, who was always very independent – after all, this would be a whole new world for him.

A local care company were brought in and the home care visits commenced. Dad had the maximum of four visits allowed per day, but these were only half-hour visits. In my view, this is one failing of today's care system. Four short visits per day where carers are supposed to feed and provide all the care required does not fit the bill for the majority of dementia sufferers as they need medication, feeding support and assistance with household tasks, but, most importantly, they need love. This is the main reason why I want people to read our story of the ways of the care system and to be aware and familiar of the procedures and protocol.

Our story

What we were not expecting was that more than 16 carers in the first week of care had been allocated to my father, and a large group of people collecting for the Red Cross to descend on my father's doorstep. They all wore red t-shirts; well, this was like waving a red flag to a bull when my father saw this large group of people at the top of our street.

When Dad just got used to a person making him a sandwich, they would zip away never to be seen again. 'Oh, my gracious,' my children would say! Dementia sufferers need continuity and reassurance.

I think I would have reacted in the same way. There was no continuity; young carers, a young girl, older carers, a motorcyclist carer, who was actually such a lovely lad, but that's exactly it – he was a lad. He did build up a rapport with my Dad, but then he disappeared and made way for a strapping man covered in tattoos and wearing shorts! A person with normal awareness may be alright with this, but not a dementia sufferer. It really was getting like a stage circus show. Wayne arrived and he genuinely wanted to bring Dad some Frank Sinatra DVDs, but Dad was very sceptical by now after having a great trail of various new strange faces and characters and ended up twirling his army baton and poking himself in the eye!! So to A&E it was. We were just grateful that it wasn't Wayne poked in his eye, who was a lovely, caring person. Well, Dad came home from hospital once again and had a course of antibiotics and the eye began to heal. A distraught Wayne came back to the house the following evening, but we felt it safer to send him away and Dad happily snoozed. Over the following few weeks, I returned home from work one day to see a young carer from a local agency leave Dad's house and I asked if everything was alright. She replied, 'Yes, I have left him a hot dinner in the lounge as he was upstairs and told me to go away!

So I thought it best I should go in, so I went straight into the house and checked. I saw Dad had fallen by his bed and was left lying in an awkward, contorted position. I quickly rang an ambulance and my lovely neighbour, Verline, who worked in the local hospital was just returning home from work. I called to her in distress and am thankful to this day that she helped me make Dad safe. Paramedics arrived and luckily, Dad was taken into the main hospital.

Tough times
After a very stressful time with my lasting power of attorney, overlooked by local authority and hospital, we managed to get Dad back home with a live-in carer package. I was immediately asked to look for care homes, although this was really going against my father's wishes. After having seen his sister suffer with a broken leg in a home in Nottingham, he always said, 'Please don't ever let me go in a home.'

For me and my husband, it has been a very prolonged battle. We did find, after much searching, two saving-grace people which I have dedicated another chapter to in the book. These are, sadly now, the late Leah Ashby from the Welsh branch of Alzheimer's Society Advocacy, and Rodger Garrett from SSAFA. Thanks to these inspiring, dedicated people who became friends. I will dearly love these two forever; without them, none of this would have been possible!

You are not alone
Please, whoever you are, and whatever age, do not feel you have to deal with hospital situations or local authority decision-making on your own. When loved ones are suffering – and I truly mean whole families here – always seek an advocate if things do not feel right, or you feel under pressure to make decisions often

under pressure due to bed blocking (where hospitals need to move patients along to make space). The system fails when it corners people to make decisions which are rushed and are not always to the best advantage of the individuals concerned.

Myself and my husband were almost forced to put Dad into care and I was in tears on this decision-making day for Dad to be released from hospital. We met an amazing manager called Wendy through a company called Helping Hands who gave us valuable advice regarding hospital equipment and was really liked by Dad as she was from our area. Wendy would say you are supposed to have a hospital bed for people being nursed at home and you are entitled to this and other things. From the very beginning of Dad's health demise with dementia, I had a live-in carer in mind as I knew this would be the only way forward to keep Dad at home. We had two young children and we also lived next door, so our situation was very different than it is for families living some distance away. Then we found Leah Ashby, advocate from the Alzheimer's Society, Wales, who had remained a close friend, and we loved her for that support and advice.

Chapter 3
Finding a live-in carer

Live-in carer stories

During the time my father spent in hospital to recover from his fall, I decided to do my own research on live-in carers. The first and foremost was always live-in care agencies. To my surprise, most of the live-in care available was only from companies away from Wales. The fees were extortionate, ranging from ridiculous hourly rates with live-in care daily rates of £85 to over £135. Most agencies have carers photographed looking adoringly into the eyes of the patient – please don't be fooled by these pictures. Check the qualifications of the carer as some undertake very short, hourly training courses which do not meet the UK Health and Safety Standards.

Unfortunately, being very green to this area of care, we did experience the good, bad and, shall I say, unusual. This is why I am writing this book to, hopefully, educate what is a growing number of people in the world of dementia care.

Our first hospital-to-home care agency was excellent with a very supportive manager called Wendy, who was there every step of the way to bring my father home with suitable care. It was an agency I was lucky to find by Google research. Dad's first live-in carer was called Maz. We were sent a photograph and breakdown of her career within the care industry. Dad had just come home from the local hospital and was sitting in his chair. At this stage, I must emphasise, Dad was able to walk, although extremely slowly. Frames were recommended, but he constantly declined them. This is a huge part of recognising dementia symptoms and of refusing to accept a change in situation. Whilst totally normal, it can be frustrating for loved ones.

Maz had arrived and was glamorous with gorgeous designer glasses, but was slightly loud and bubbly. The first greeting to my father was, 'Oh, aren't you lucky to have all these women around you.' Wendy was also at the house to see all was ok. She did say, while winking at me, 'On that note, I'm leaving. See you soon.' That was the last greeting Dad really needed to hear as, being a very proud man, it was not really the best way of an introduction to him.

I would advise anyone to go with a hospital-to-home agency to begin with as they are very supportive. Wendy did explain Dad should be entitled to certain hospital equipment such as a special bed and mattress. This we did not get on Dad's first time home, but he was able to walk slightly then. Maz was a good cook and certainly lightened the load with her nursing skills, although Dad could get a little demanding with some outbursts.

After two weeks, it was time for Maz to return to her family. It had been a little difficult at times with a carer who had a strong New Zealand accent, and it is worth being aware that strange accents can be difficult for dementia sufferers as they are not familiar to them.

Our next carer from the agency was Steve, who was a lovely person and had previously been a monk. Although he was an obliging young carer, he did enjoy walking about without shoes. This used to annoy Dad, as did the serving of meals on a plate still in a plastic container. Steve was also partial to a spring onion, alone on a plate, for his tea, which used to perplex us all. This was the first of many unusual experiences of live-in carers.

What is important here is that, although agencies can have all the correct training and qualifications listed of their carers, together with their experience, which look great on paper, it is not always the case. With dementia constantly increasing, and even young people suffering from stroke which can lead to dementia, it is of vital importance that we get it right. I do feel that all agencies should put carers through their paces come what may, including being shown how to dress correctly, being courteous and having the correct knowledge of domiciliary duties which are checked and monitored. One carer, who came from South Africa, had only completed a half day of hoist training. This came to light after a hoist injury my Dad received on Boxing Day, which is explained later in the book. This is why all carers should be checked regularly; after all, we have moderators and verifiers for nursery care, schools, colleges and universities.

Impeccable care should also be scrutinised and vetted at regular intervals, particularly since there are some carers coming through the system who are looking after our loved ones and not coming up to task! Care and nursing homes are rigorously examined and this, I believe, should also be the case for live-in carers who are, realistically, in a more vulnerable situation.

The normal timescale with agencies of live-in care can be from two weeks to two months, depending mainly on financial constraints and care required. When Steve had completed two weeks we were then sent a lady from South Africa called Muriel who was a great carer, albeit a little loud. This, once again, was good for short-term care. Whilst care was better with a live-in carer to ensure there was someone with my father at all times, myself and my husband would cover the carers' breaks which were usually 2 hours per day. This was quite nice as it was great to have more quality time with Dad, and he loved spending time with his grandchildren.

More local care

Whilst care had now been in place for a couple of months, it was very expensive and I began to look at reducing costs and finding a local agency. This took some research, but I eventually found magnificent carers. They were based in Wales, which was a huge bonus, and did look exactly what we were looking for. As with the majority of agencies their charges were based on a three-tier system, ranging from basic companionship care, to more demanding personal care and domiciliary duties, to PEG feeds and high-end care. The general form took place with a visit from a couple of managers who were very nice and keen that Dad should have a glass of sherry with his meals. They were a little more interested in the more refined elements which, now, I think is good, but let's get down to basics every time: good empathy, care and cleaning! It certainly was not a time to be playing Candy Crush, which is what we experienced with a few live-in carers, when on duty of care!

It is important to note that all agencies charge a basic fee and then set you up with a package to suit. Although help is available through various local authorities, there is always a top-up fee to pay unless its continued health care, which is nursing care and a different thing altogether. There is more detail on this at the end of the book.

Chapter 4

Dream to nightmare!

To be honest, sometimes you are in a corner with care as, when you need someone desperately, you have very little choice.

At first, a lovely local agency seemed to answer our prayers of meeting the needs of my father. We were introduced by a phone call to Lorna, a South African lady, who seemed very nice: really calm and well spoken.

She arrived and parked her car outside and we thought, *Great, a carer who can drive.* When I first met her I noticed she walked incredibly slowly due to very bad knees and I did question if she should be in the care profession.

Lorna came in and was introduced to Dad; this was the start of several introductions to carers. At first, Lorna seemed lovely and got on with washing and enjoyed preparing food which was great. On the first weekend she was with us we had a wedding to attend and were so thankful that Dad had a good carer.

One thing which did concern me was that she mentioned her husband would be coming over to England and could he call and see her. I was slightly concerned at this because, professionally, carers are not supposed to have people to the house, but I thought a quick meeting with Lorna would be fine and I arranged for a few of Dad's friends to call, which was a godsend.

We went to my cousin's wedding and had a good time. This was a good thing, as we didn't know what would be in store over the next two weeks. The next morning, I received a text from one of Dad's friends saying he was concerned that the carer had her husband with her on the Saturday for the whole duration of his visit to see Dad and didn't think this was the way it should be. When I saw her the next day, she explained that Dad had been left in his chair all night as he didn't want to be moved. At this time, Dad was walking, but he was unsteady. From then onwards, we noticed a lot. My husband went in most evenings to assist Lorna, yet she would sit on the top stair and watch my husband help get Dad ready for night time. Dad's condition could make things difficult with him not consenting to care, but we muddled through, and although things seemed to be just OK, we were always concerned as he seemed to be upset with Lorna.

On her time off, I chaperoned her to my hair salon for a trim and wondered why didn't she drive anywhere. She said she needed to tax her car and that it also needed work completed on it, so the following week her husband would appear again to swap cars! She did say, in front of my children in the car, that Dad was extremely difficult. I had to ask her to kindly refrain from talking about Dad's care in front of the children.

I finally rang the agency to speak with a manager when, once again, she was extremely fierce with Dad whilst she was getting him ready. We had an engineer out to fix the brand new washing machine and he told us that the water tap had been turned off on the water outlet. At this stage, I knew we had to get a new carer on board.

When I contacted the agency, the manager was really quite defensive of Lorna and couldn't, and wouldn't, believe what had gone on. At this time of writing we put it down to a bad experience and eventually, after another visit from the agency, the owners were understanding and said Lorna should never have put us in the position of being expected to have her husband on duty and this was a concern. I guess desperate times requires desperate measures.

Fairly quickly, the agency sent us another lady who was local but had been working across the bridge. Again she sounded amazing on the phone and seemed to have looked after several people with dementia. Her name was Mary and she was young, but very good with Dad and made him all the food he loved, including sardines on toast and traditional food. When I first met Mary I thought she looked like she was only in her early forties and did not like your 'typical' carer, but by now we had met a wide range of people. The only problem was that she liked to go away for longer breaks and this was a concern for us as we have a young family and required carers to get on with the care and not have us stressing about their attendance and Dad's care.

Mary was with us for a good few weeks and I learned some interesting facts. One evening, Mary held up a patterned pair of pyjamas and Dad cried out, 'Oh, not pennies from heaven,' Mary explained that dementia sufferers only like plain items as patterns can confuse them, hence the title of the book being born. Although a good carer, Dad did show signs of aggression now and then as she would talk about him in front of him. It is wrong for carers looking after someone with dementia as it is rude for anyone, but her knowledge was good in other areas. Mary also could talk for England, Ireland, Scotland and Wales and, once again, we just wanted Dad cared for without all the concern of myself or husband returning into our family home late for no reason.

Mary was due to have a break after her three weeks and Dad had taken a turn with his health on the commencement of a cover carer from a different agency as we found the present agency could not accommodate us with a relief carer. On the day Mary was due to go on a break and return after one week, Dad had a UTI. A new carer, called Nadia, from another agency turned up with about ten black bags full of pillows and items and three huge cases. She was Romanian and really sweet. When she went to settle in the room at handover stage, which is common in all care, I could hear the mutterings of Mary wishing her all the best and over egging the situation regarding Dad's temperament. At the same time she was saying he isn't good at all really now and in my experience he should have been turned away from the side he was lying on as he had cellulitis in the elbow, which we later found out. To be honest, I felt a little violated and felt that she should be minding her own business, but at the same time wanting to welcome Nadia. To make matters worse, the new agency had booked Nadia as a permanent carer for six weeks, which was a complete mistake, and Maria explained she was due back in one week's time. We were looking at carers who really could do a week on and off but this was proving difficult with all agencies.

At this time my mind was clocking over that we should advertise ourselves for private carers. Which we later did, to our advantage.

Chapter 5
Hospital again and complete despair

The day after Mary had left for her break, Nadia thought Dad looked unwell and kept saying to my husband and myself that she thought it was a mistake for us to look after Dad at home, saying, 'He is too unwell and you need to get on with your lives.' She told us that in Romania dementia care was superb and we should think of that.

I couldn't work this out. Nadia was here telling us this and yet she was in this country working. My Dad was ill, but surely he could have medication to help him? I even started questioning myself. The start of six months of really low times was about to happen and none of it was to be of our making.

The following morning, Dad was admitted to University Hospital of Wales in Cardiff and a severe urinary tract infection (UTI) and cellulitis was diagnosed. Myself and my husband thought Dad would be given a course of antibiotics and would be home again. That wasn't the case.

When I went to see him the day he was admitted to the assessment unit he was totally confused and in a deep, almost transient, state. I now know this was the result of the UTI. They are the most awful infections when people are elderly and need immediate antibiotics to alleviate the condition. However, when I asked to see Dad's notes from the hospital I was refused and looked at quite judgementally. It was the first time I felt a sick feeling inside, and there were many of these to follow.

Dad had a few sores, which were questioned. Carers reported he would sometimes knock himself, but these subsequently healed. However, Dad had cellulitis in his elbow and this was being treated as it can be dangerous if it spreads. In Dad's case, he had been in the same position for too long and I felt the carers should have been rotating him. However, I appreciate it can be difficult to move a patient, but when it is necessary for their well-being it must be done.

After a couple of days, Dad was moved to a dementia ward and nursed back to health and improved after a normal couple of weeks. The sad thing is that he went into hospital with the ability to walk, although unsteady on his feet. He remained in hospital for six needless months, due to the instigation of a POVA (protection of a vulnerable adult), together with a DoLS assessment.

During this time, I had also contacted Mary and she said she was ready to come back to look after Dad. I had a gut feeling we would never hear from her again as some of the carers before her. To some it is merely doing a job, but not for all, as I explain later.

How my stomach still turns as I write that. It made me feel cruel, wrong and all the worst things an only daughter can feel when doing her best, with her husband, to keep their Dad home and safe. My tears are actually building up as I think about what we have been through …

Looking back, I can safely say that a POVA is quite normal to help protect vulnerable adults; however, at the time I think we were also vulnerable, but the system does not allow for that.

Chapter 6

Saving graces and inner strengths

Since losing my mother on Christmas Day in 1982, and always being a strong person inside, I was always ten steps ahead in my mind when thinking of looking after my father. After a short break for a few days with my husband and children whilst Dad got stronger and was in safe hands, I thought of all wrongdoings that had gone on and kept a diary, as my mum had done with her care.

On return from our short break, I kept asking when and why Dad was not being released from hospital. It felt, to me, like a life sentence. We learned that the discharge liaison officer and social worker were away. These are, apparently, normal occurrences in hospital, but they do us, and our loved ones, no favours whatsoever.

I tried to make the best of the situation and even bought a wheelchair from the British Red Cross, who were fantastic, as I would have had a long wait for a hospital one. We took Dad out to the hospital coffee shop and cafe. He was happy in himself as he enjoyed seeing people. After a month, I contacted the Alzheimer's Advocacy service in Cardiff where I met Leah Ashby, our saving grace. Leah was told everything about Dad's position and, unfortunately, made us aware that it is not uncommon and many elderly sufferers get admitted to hospital from falls or illnesses with the majority ending up in care homes, there being no choice or family to look after them.

In our case, there had been several wrong doings by the hospital and others involved in the planning of Dad's care. Finally, prior to Dad's hospital discharge meeting, we had a meeting where a social worker declared to us he would not be coming home as there was not sufficient care for him and advising that he needed elderly mental health care in a care home. He suggested we start looking for one immediately.

My lasting power of attorney (LPOA) was ignored. Incorrect information was looked at for the meeting – the list went on!

Leah advised the social worker I had LPOA and launched an enquiry herself into the way we had been treated. I do not wish for anyone to have to go through what we went through – it was appalling.

Please investigate paying for a LPAO, Health and Welfare and Finance, as it gives you the power to make the choice in the best interests of a loved one. However, it must be done early prior to any illnesses setting in.

Moving forward, I did look into care packages and the only valid way to look after my father would be, as we planned, with a live-in carer. However, from hospital to home, I planned to advertise for Dad's specific needs and this was to be a priority.

The final discharge meeting was underway and after several frosty-faced liaison workers, I had a carer booked for Dad's homecoming on December 5th 2014.

Chapter 7
Bring him home

After my husband playing Alfie Boe's "Bring him home" on several occasions, Dad was eventually home, safe with a hospital bed and hoist in place. I understand all these things take time, but after all the worry it was relief tinged with concern for getting it completely right with care. These things don't come overnight. No matter how many leaflets or advisors you get given, the only way to experience it is by going through it. In fact, we have learned so much about care, various systems and agencies we feel like we could train people in it.

I have spent many hours researching and holding meetings and speaking with Leah and others that I have absorbed so much information. I provide many contacts and associations at the end of this book to hopefully help others going through a similar situation.

A huge difference this time was that we had an agency involved with Dad's many needs. Carewatch (now Pineshield) have been a tremendous support to us. The majority of carers were men, but also some women, and they have shown us how great care can be. We did have another local agency who were not as experienced and professional with many barely youngsters just out of school. I strongly believe that you cannot expect a really young, inexperienced female, or male, to perform personal care duties when they just have basic knowledge in dealing with dementia conditions of which there are actually over 80 types.

Dad had been home for almost three weeks with live-in carer Tamara from New Zealand. She was attentive and a very nice person, but did keep calling Dad "grandad" and I think this made Dad a bit confused. It was a really unfortunate incident which showed us she really did not have the qualifications recognised in this country for hoisting.

Things had been going well until Boxing Day and early after breakfast I went into see Dad with my daughter, who was age eight at the time. Dad was with Tamara and the agency carer ready to be set up for the day. I heard a dreadful yelp from Dad and rushed into the lounge only to see the most horrific sight.

Both carers were in a right mess; they had tried to hoist Dad onto a sofa, the hoist had clobbered Dad on his head and the actual metal frame was practically on top of him and the carer. I quickly yelled ice, my daughter brought me an ice pack, the agency carer was saying sorry repeatedly. I can't believe how I kept calm after saying, 'What the hell are you both doing?'

Tamara looked ashen and did not know what to say. In the meantime, all jokes aside, Dad's head looked like it was from a cartoon with a huge lump growing on it. I thought this is the end. I could not believe it. I rang an ambulance and Dad's carer, who was due to go on her week off break, was ready to pack and leave. I said to her, 'I want you to go with Dad to the hospital, please.' The agency carer practically ran away from the house. Say no more. Tamara completed an accident form.

Once again, I felt sick thinking, *Dad's been in hospital for six months, I'll never see him again.* Thank goodness he was sent home the same night, to our huge relief. We were told there were no beds and were just grateful he was home.

Needless to say, there was another investigation into this most serious of incidents and this is where it was uncovered that the agency staff did not communicate correctly with the live-in carer and both were really blaming each other. The live-in carer was not sufficiently certified. Both have not been seen or heard of since.

Privately advertised care

A whole new chapter was to begin with a sense of calm at last.

I had advertised for private carers, preferably local. I did this in the local press and received a great response.

The rule of thumb when interviewing and advertising for live-in carers is to explain carefully about the person they are looking after and most definitely make sure that legal checks and qualifications are in place plus experience and references. It is a huge responsibility as the carer and person they care for must be able to get on and after a few live-in carers, we found gold after, shall I say, the bronze.

The first live-in carer I interviewed was nice enough, although after a couple of months Dad was showing signs of not being too happy with them. We felt they had no empathy with our children and, after seeing a few things, we decided to advertise again. We found a wonderful local carer who had the most lovely way with her. Dad's care was impeccable, the trouble was she was missing being away from her boyfriend, so, after a couple of months, we were left once again with the power of advertising. I have to say now, looking back, it was most definitely worth every bad moment to eventually begin to get it right and, wow, we certainly did. Friends and family would say, 'You are doing so well, how do you do it?' To be honest, I think to honour my Dad's wishes was the empowering thing for us to keep him home safe with the family he loved, and having his grandchildren close each day – who could possibly ask for more?

To this day, I will always remember interviewing Nathalie, Adam and Sabina. Sabina was heaven sent as she lived locally, was qualified to the hilt and Dad loved her. We all do, to this day.

Sabina was taken on to help with Dad's care with the live-in carers. Nathalie was amazing, she was so thorough – a little pocket rocket. She was so dedicated that even when she became ill, she made Dad a special, hand-knitted cushion with all zips and buttons. Dad would spend hours doing buttons up and keeping busy. When Nathalie had time, whilst Dad slept, she wrote out impeccable details of what Dad's needs were for future carers. This had really helped them.

I would come home from work to find Nathalie dancing and singing with Dad whilst he also told her off if she missed cleaning a bit of glass on the lighting. We would all laugh and have family time. Nathalie also enjoyed cooking.

Chapter 8

Saving the best until last!

After about five months, sadly, Nathalie had to move to England to help her own family, but she wrote us a beautiful card which I will always treasure. She was a gold-standard carer.

It was in August when Adam had taken our main live-in carer role with Nathalie and together they were a fab team. Adam, to this day, as our final two carers, will always be like family. We spent summers having barbecues and taking Dad out to friends' garden parties – he had a lovely time and enjoyed listening to Elaine Paige on a Sunday with Adam who loves all music. The children used to enjoy playing when Adam was looking after Pops. They would tease him to give extra biscuits, but that was ok as Pops loved those days too!

Adam learnt how to cook a great fish finger sandwich which Dad loved and we would both took Pops out for a coffee on the Green Links bus which was also a godsend. This was a transport service available for a very small joining fee and would pick up wheelchair users, or other people, and enable them to enjoy everyday, normal events.

Rodger and Leah would call in to see Pops, and all of us, and he would enjoy seeing our familiar friend who had contributed so much support to having us keep Dad home.

Our new carer, to work weekly shifts on and off with Adam, was Angela. Formerly from a good nursing home in Penarth, Angela was amazing. She was so caring with Dad, was lovely natured and amazing with nursing care as Dad was slowly becoming a little more in need of support with eating and drinking.

Carers would have his favourite music on and he would look through books and photograph albums and his friends, Mike, Ken and others, would love to call in and see him for a catch-up.

Dad also loved looking at the garden and watching the birds and some squirrels. Angela enjoyed putting food out for the birds and they would sit and watch for hours. It was great to see your loved one in their own home in familiar surroundings and know they are safe. It makes me feel all warm and happy to remember this and I feel very proud. The one person who I haven't mentioned is my husband Jason, and throughout the whole chapter of Dad's life – pre-, with and after – he has been my rock, my support. If a person doesn't have that close family help, it is going to be a tough ride. He stepped in at the last minute on many occasions and was wonderful in supporting my Dad's care at home.

When Angela went on maternity leave, we were very fortunate she had recommended a friend, Nam, who had worked alongside her in the nursing home in Penarth. Nam was wonderful – full of fun and a joy to have around. Dad loved her dancing and joking with him, taking his cap and then flicking it around. Adam, Nam, Angela and Sabina were the best carers from the heart that anyone could wish for.

After three years at home, my Dad passed away with his family and carers around him. I do feel proud of him and all of us for enabling him to have a happy last few years at home where he wanted to be.

Dance, Dance, Wherever You May Be!

Live

Useful Contacts for Carers and Family Members

During the writing of my book there have been many useful websites and contact numbers and I have tried to give a large selection here as a handy guide.

Alzheimer's Association, The Strand, London   02078 632444

Alzheimer's Society - Cardiff and The Vale

Supports people with dementia, their families and carers.

Ty Hapus, Holton Rd   01446 738024

Oldwell Court in Penylan   02920 434960

Cardiff and Vale (UHB)   02920 745692

Local Authority   01446 700111

Age Connect, Wales   02922 400029

Help with services for older people, nail cutting, social activities, Good Neighbour scheme.

www.age-concern-cardiff.org.uk

Advocacy Support Cymru   02920 540444

Age Cymru   0800 0223444

or advice@agecymru.org.uk

Armed Forces Community Covenant   02920 872087

For veterans, serving members of the Armed Forces and their families for concern.

British Red Cross   07921 404327

Provide a number of services including equipment for elderly people.

Mobility Aids Service   08444 122756

Local Authorities will have transport help and other numbers to aid people and their carers to get about to activities and appointments.

SSAFA   02920 383852

Armed Forces Charity https://www.ssafa.org.uk

Admiral Nurses   0800 8886678

Lightning Source UK Ltd.
Milton Keynes UK
UKOW06f0402261017
311645UK00006B/320/P